THE COMPLETE KETO DIET COOKBOOK

THE BEST RECIPES THAT WILL HELP YOU LOSE WEIGHT, BALANCE HORMONES, BOOST BRAIN HEALTH AND REVERSE DISEASE

THE COD PRESS

TABLE OF CONTENTS:

CHAPTER 1: BREAKFAST RECIPES 4

    CREPES WITH SPINACH, BACON AND MUSHROOM FILLING 5
    ZUCCHINI NUT COOKIES 8
    BERRY NUT AND SEED CRUNCH 10
    BACON STUFFED AVOCADOS 12
    ROASTED ASPARAGUS WITH LEMON AND GOAT CHEESE 14
    AVOCADO GREEK OMELET 16
    TUNA MELT WITH EGG 18
    CHORIZO STUFFED BELL PEPPERS 20
    EASY SHAKSHUKA 22
    MEDITERRANEAN-TWIST SALMON 24

CHAPTER 2: MEAT RECIPES 27

    SAUSAGE BAKE 28
    STUFFED AND ROLLED PORK TENDERLOIN 30
    SWEET AND SOUR FAUX MEAT BALLS 33
    CHEESEBURGER QUESADILLAS 35
    BEEF BULGOGI 38
    PRESSURE COOKER CHUCK ROAST WITH VEGGIES AND GRAVY 40
    BACON-WRAPPED DOUBLE DOGS 42
    SESAME SAKE PORK MEDALLIONS 44
    BALSAMIC ROASTED BRUSSELS SPROUTS WITH BACON 46
    ITALIAN MINI MEAT LOAVES 48

CHAPTER 3: FISH & SEAFOOD RECIPES 52

    BELL PEPPER AND LEMON SALMON 53
    BAKED HADDOCK 55
    SHRIMP AND VEGGIE STUFFED ZUCCHINI 57

CHAPTER 4: VEGETABLE RECIPES 61

    EGGPLANT GRATIN 62
    GRILLED BROCCOLI RABE 64
    BAKED MASHED PARSNIPS 66

ROASTED VEGETABLES WITH SPAGHETTI SQUASH	68
HALLOUMI PARMIGIANA	72
HABANERO COOKIES	75
VEGETARIAN SPINACH AND MUSHROOM ENCHILADAS	77
VEGAN BLUEBERRY MUFFINS	80

CHAPTER 5: SNACK & APPETIZERS RECIPES 83

BACON-WRAPPED STUFFED MUSHROOMS	84
BAKED WALNUTS	86
BACON-WRAPPED MEATLOAF	88
TURNIP BAKE	90
SAUSAGE-STUFFED PIQUILLO PEPPERS	92
ROASTED GREEN BEANS AND SHALLOTS	94
ROASTED RADISHES WITH ONIONS	96
SPICY RANCH CAULIFLOWER CRACKERS	98
SIMPLE BRITISH FLAPJACK	100
BACON-BLEU CHEESE BALL	102

CHAPTER 6: POULTRY RECIPES 105

CHICKEN PAPRIKA	106
PRETZEL CHICKEN DIPPERS	108
CHICKEN KABOBS	110

© Copyright 2021 by The Cod Press All rights reserved.

The following Book is reproduced below with the goal of providing information that is as accurate and reliable as possible. Regardless, purchasing this Book can be seen as consent to the fact that both the publisher and the author of this book are in no way experts on the topics discussed within and that any recommendations or suggestions that are made herein are for entertainment purposes only. Professionals should be consulted as needed prior to undertaking any of the action endorsed herein.

This declaration is deemed fair and valid by both the American Bar Association and the Committee of Publishers Association and is legally binding throughout the United States.

Furthermore, the transmission, duplication, or reproduction of any of the following work including specific information will be considered an illegal act irrespective of if it is done electronically or in print. This extends to creating a secondary or tertiary copy of the work or a recorded copy and is only allowed with the express written consent from the Publisher. All additional right reserved.

The information in the following pages is broadly considered a truthful and accurate account of facts and as such, any inattention, use, or misuse of the information in question by the reader will render any resulting actions solely under their purview. There are no scenarios in which the publisher or the original author of this work can be in any fashion deemed liable for any hardship or damages that may befall them after undertaking information described herein.

Additionally, the information in the following pages is intended only for informational purposes and should thus be thought of as universal. As befitting its nature, it is presented without assurance regarding its prolonged validity or interim quality. Trademarks that are mentioned are done without written consent and can in no way be considered an endorsement from the trademark holder.

CHAPTER 1:

BREAKFAST RECIPES

CREPES WITH SPINACH, BACON AND MUSHROOM FILLING

Prep:
35 mins
Cook:
20 mins
Additional:
10 mins
Total:
1 hr 5 mins
Servings:
4
Yield:
4 servings

INGREDIENTS:

1 recipe Basic Crepes
6 slices bacon
1 tablespoon unsalted butter
½ pound fresh mushrooms, sliced
3 tablespoons unsalted butter
¼ cup all-purpose flour
1 cup milk
1 (10 ounce) package frozen chopped spinach, thawed and drained
1 tablespoon chopped fresh parsley

2 tablespoons grated Parmesan cheese
salt and pepper to taste
⅔ cup chicken broth
2 eggs
½ cup lemon juice
salt and pepper to taste

DIRECTIONS:

1

Prepare Basic Crepes recipe according to recipe directions. Separate with wax paper and keep warm until ready to serve.

2

Place bacon in a large, deep skillet. Cook over medium-high heat until evenly brown. Drain, crumble and set aside. Reserve about 1 tablespoon drippings, add 1 tablespoon butter, and saute mushrooms.

3

In a separate saucepan, melt 3 tablespoons butter over medium heat. Whisk in 1/4 cup flour, stirring constantly, until a smooth paste is formed. Gradually stir in 1 cup milk, stirring constantly until a smooth thick gravy is formed. Add bacon, mushrooms, spinach, parsley, Parmesan cheese, salt and pepper. Let cook until somewhat thick, about 10 minutes.

4

In saucepan bring broth to a boil. In a small bowl, whisk together eggs and lemon juice. Temper eggs and broth together whisking constantly so as to cook, but not to scramble the eggs. (Cooking eggs to 170 degrees F). Again, salt and pepper to taste.

5
Fill each crepe with spinach and meat filling, roll up, and top with warm egg sauce.

NUTRITION FACTS:

445 calories; protein 15.9g; carbohydrates 17.9g; fat 35.6g; cholesterol 160mg;

ZUCCHINI NUT COOKIES

Prep:
15 mins
Cook:
15 mins
Additional:
30 mins
Total:
1 hr
Servings:
36
Yield:
3 dozen

INGREDIENTS:

½ cup packed brown sugar
½ cup white sugar
½ cup shortening
1 egg
2 cups sifted all-purpose flour
1 teaspoon baking soda
1 teaspoon ground cinnamon
½ teaspoon ground nutmeg
½ teaspoon ground cloves
¼ teaspoon salt
1 cup grated zucchini
1 cup raisins
½ cup chopped walnuts

DIRECTIONS:

1

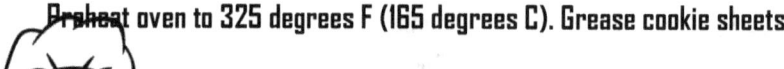Preheat oven to 325 degrees F (165 degrees C). Grease cookie sheets.

2

Cream together shortening, brown sugar, and white sugar until smooth. Beat in egg. Combine the flour, baking soda, salt, cinnamon, nutmeg, and cloves; stir into the creamed mixture. Mix in zucchini, raisins, and walnuts. Drop by rounded tablespoons onto the prepared baking sheets.

3

Bake 15 minutes in the preheated oven, or until lightly browned. Cool on the cookie sheets for a few minutes before removing to wire racks to cool completely.

NUTRITION FACTS:

99 calories; protein 1.3g; carbohydrates 14.7g; fat 4.2g; cholesterol 5.2mg; sodium 54.9mg.

BERRY NUT AND SEED CRUNCH

Prep:
10 mins
Cook:
10 mins
Additional:
30 mins
Total:
50 mins
Servings:
16
Yield:
16 servings

INGREDIENTS:

½ cup brown sugar
1 ½ cups walnuts
2 tablespoons sesame seeds
1 cup hulled pumpkin seeds
1 cup sunflower seeds
¾ cup raspberry-flavored dried cranberries

DIRECTIONS:

1

Line a baking sheet with parchment paper.

2

Heat brown sugar in a saucepan over medium-low heat until melted; stir in walnuts and sesame seeds until walnuts are coated with sugar and sesame seeds. Transfer coated walnuts to the prepared baking sheet; set aside until cooled.

3

Mix coated walnuts, pumpkin seeds, sunflower seeds, and cranberries together in a bowl.

NUTRITION FACTS:

213 calories; protein 5.9g; carbohydrates 14.2g; fat 16.5g;

BACON STUFFED AVOCADOS

Prep:
10 mins
Cook:
20 mins
Total:
30 mins
Servings:
8
Yield:
8 avocado halves

INGREDIENTS:

8 slices bacon
½ cup butter
¼ cup brown sugar
¼ cup red wine vinegar
1 tablespoon soy sauce
2 cloves garlic, chopped
salt to taste
4 avocados - halved, pitted, and peeled

DIRECTIONS:

1

Place bacon in a large
skillet and cook over medium-high heat,
turning occasionally,
until evenly browned, about 10 minutes.
Drain bacon slices on paper towels; crumble.

2

Mix butter, brown sugar, vinegar, soy sauce, and garlic in a saucepan; cook and stir mixture over medium heat until sugar is dissolved, about 10 minutes.

3

Sprinkle avocado halves with salt; fill each half with crumbled bacon. Drizzle sauce over filled avocados.

NUTRITION FACTS:

3 calories; protein 5.7g; carbohydrates 14.1g; fat 30.1g; cholesterol 40.5mg;

ROASTED ASPARAGUS WITH LEMON AND GOAT CHEESE

Prep:
10 mins
Additional:
20 mins
Total:
30 mins
Servings:
6
Yield:
6 servings

INGREDIENTS:

2 pounds fresh asparagus, trimmed
1 tablespoon olive oil
½ cup Swanson® Vegetable Broth
3 ounces soft goat cheese, crumbled
1 tablespoon lemon juice
1 teaspoon grated lemon zest

DIRECTIONS:

1

Set the oven to 425 degrees F. Spray a roasting pan with vegetable cooking spray.

2

Stir the asparagus and oil in the pan. Season the asparagus as desired. Add the broth.

3

Roast the asparagus for 20 minutes or until tender, stirring once during cooking. Top with the cheese, lemon juice and lemon zest.

NUTRITION FACTS:

104 calories; protein 6.4g; carbohydrates 6.8g; fat 6.7g; cholesterol 11.2mg; sodium 154.5mg.

AVOCADO GREEK OMELET

Prep:
15 mins
Cook:
8 mins
Total:
23 mins
Servings:
2
Yield:
1 omelet

INGREDIENTS:

3 eggs
¾ cup feta cheese
½ avocado, diced
½ cup diced tomatoes
¼ cup chopped Kalamata olives
1 tablespoon chopped fresh basil

DIRECTIONS:

1

Whisk eggs in a small bowl until smooth.

2

Preheat a nonstick skillet over medium heat. Pour in eggs. Scatter feta cheese, avocado, tomatoes, olives, and basil over 1 side. Cook until bottom is golden brown, about 5 minutes. Fold over; cook until center is set, about 3 minutes more.

NUTRITION FACTS:

392 calories; protein 19.1g; carbohydrates 10.5g; fat 31.3g; cholesterol 329.1mg;

TUNA MELT WITH EGG

Prep:
25 mins
Cook:
5 mins
Total:
30 mins
Servings:
6
Yield:
6 tuna melts

INGREDIENTS:

2 (5 ounce) cans water-packed tuna, drained
1 cup mayonnaise
¼ cup finely chopped celery
¼ cup finely chopped green onions
¼ cup finely chopped carrots
2 hard-boiled eggs, chopped
8 large ripe olives, sliced
2 teaspoons Dijon mustard (such as Grey Poupon®)
¼ cup butter, melted
12 slices sourdough bread, or more to taste
12 slices Swiss cheese

DIRECTIONS:

1
Set an oven rack about 6 inches from the heat source and preheat the oven's broiler. Line a baking sheet with parchment paper.

2
Combine tuna, mayonnaise, celery, green onions, carrots, hard-boiled eggs, olives, and mustard in a bowl; mix until well combined.

3
Brush melted butter on one side of each bread slice. Top an unbuttered side with a slice of cheese, some tuna salad, another slice of cheese, and another slice of bread, buttered side facing up. Repeat with remaining ingredients. Transfer sandwiches to the prepared baking sheet.

4
Broil in the preheated oven until bread is toasted and cheese is melted, 3 to 5 minutes.

NUTRITION FACTS:

778 calories; protein 34.6g; carbohydrates 34.3g; fat 56.2g; cholesterol 169.7mg;

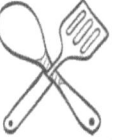

CHORIZO STUFFED BELL PEPPERS

Prep:
40 mins
Cook:
1 hr
Total:
1 hr 40 mins

INGREDIENTS:

6 bell peppers, tops cut off and seeded
1 pound chorizo sausage
1 stalk celery, minced
1 carrot, minced
½ cup chopped onion
4 cloves garlic, minced
salt and pepper to taste
1 (14.5 ounce) can whole peeled tomatoes, chopped
1 tablespoon Worcestershire sauce
chopped fresh parsley
chopped fresh basil
½ cup uncooked long grain rice
½ cup water
⅓ cup shredded Monterey Jack cheese
⅓ cup shredded Cheddar cheese
⅓ cup shredded Mozzarella Cheese
1 (10.75 ounce) can tomato soup

DIRECTIONS:

1
Bring a large pot of water to boil. Place peppers in boiling water, and cook 5 minutes. Remove, and set aside to cool.

2
Preheat oven to 350 degrees F (175 degrees C).

3
In a large skillet, cook chorizo until almost brown. Drain fat. Stir in celery, carrots, onions, and garlic. Cook until soft, about 5 minutes. Season with salt and pepper. Stir in tomatoes, Worcestershire sauce, parsley, basil, rice, and water. Cover, and simmer until rice is cooked, about 15 minutes. Remove from heat, and mix in Monterey Jack, Cheddar, and Mozzarella cheeses.

4
Place peppers upright on a baking sheet. Stuff each pepper with the chorizo mixture. Sprinkle extra cheese on top.

5
In a small bowl, combine tomato soup with just enough water to give the soup the consistency of gravy. Pour generously over peppers. Cover with foil.

6
Bake in preheated oven about 30 minutes.

NUTRITION FACTS:

559 calories; protein 27.6g; carbohydrates 33.9g;

fat 35.4g; cholesterol 82.8mg;

EASY SHAKSHUKA

Prep:
10 mins
Cook:
35 mins
Total:
45 mins
Servings:
4
Yield:
4 servings

INGREDIENTS:

1 tablespoon olive oil
2 cloves garlic, minced
1 onion, cut into 2 inch pieces
1 green bell pepper, cut into 2 inch pieces
1 (28 ounce) can whole peeled plum tomatoes with juice
1 teaspoon paprika, or to taste
2 slices pickled jalapeno pepper, finely chopped
4 eggs
4 (6 inch) pita bread (Optional)

DIRECTIONS:

1

Heat the vegetable oil in a deep skillet over medium heat. Stir in the garlic, onion, and bell pepper; cook and stir until the onion has softened and turned translucent, about 5 minutes. Add the canned tomatoes, paprika and jalapenos; stir, using the back of a spoon to break up the tomatoes. Simmer for about 25 minutes.

2

Crack an egg into a small bowl, then gently slip the egg into the tomato sauce. Repeat with the remaining eggs. Cook the eggs until the whites are firm and the yolks have thickened but are not hard, 2 1/2 to 3 minutes. If the tomato sauce gets dry, add a few tablespoons of water. Remove the eggs with a slotted spoon, place onto a warm plate, and serve with the tomato sauce and pita bread.

NUTRITION FACTS:

294 calories; protein 13.1g; carbohydrates 40.9g; fat 9.4g; cholesterol 186mg; sodium 654.2mg.

MEDITERRANEAN-TWIST SALMON

Prep:
10 mins
Cook:
20 mins
Total:
30 mins
Servings:
2
Yield:
2 servings

INGREDIENTS:

Salmon:
1 teaspoon olive oil
2 (4 ounce) fillets salmon
Sauce:
2 tablespoons olive oil
1 clove garlic, minced
½ cup chopped tomatoes, or more to taste
1 tablespoon balsamic vinegar
6 fresh basil leaves, chopped

DIRECTIONS:

1

Heat 1 teaspoon olive oil in a saucepan over medium heat. Cook salmon in the hot oil until cooked through and flakes easily with a fork, 5 to 7 minutes per side.

2

Heat 2 tablespoons olive oil in a separate saucepan over medium heat; add garlic and cook until fragrant, about 1 minute. Add tomatoes; cook until heated through, about 5 minutes. Pour balsamic vinegar into tomato mixture; add basil. Cook and stir tomato mixture until flavors blend, about 3 minutes.

3

Place salmon on a plate and top with tomato sauce.

NUTRITION FACTS:

347 calories; protein 24.8g; carbohydrates 3.8g; fat 25.6g; cholesterol 75.7mg; sodium 62.8mg.

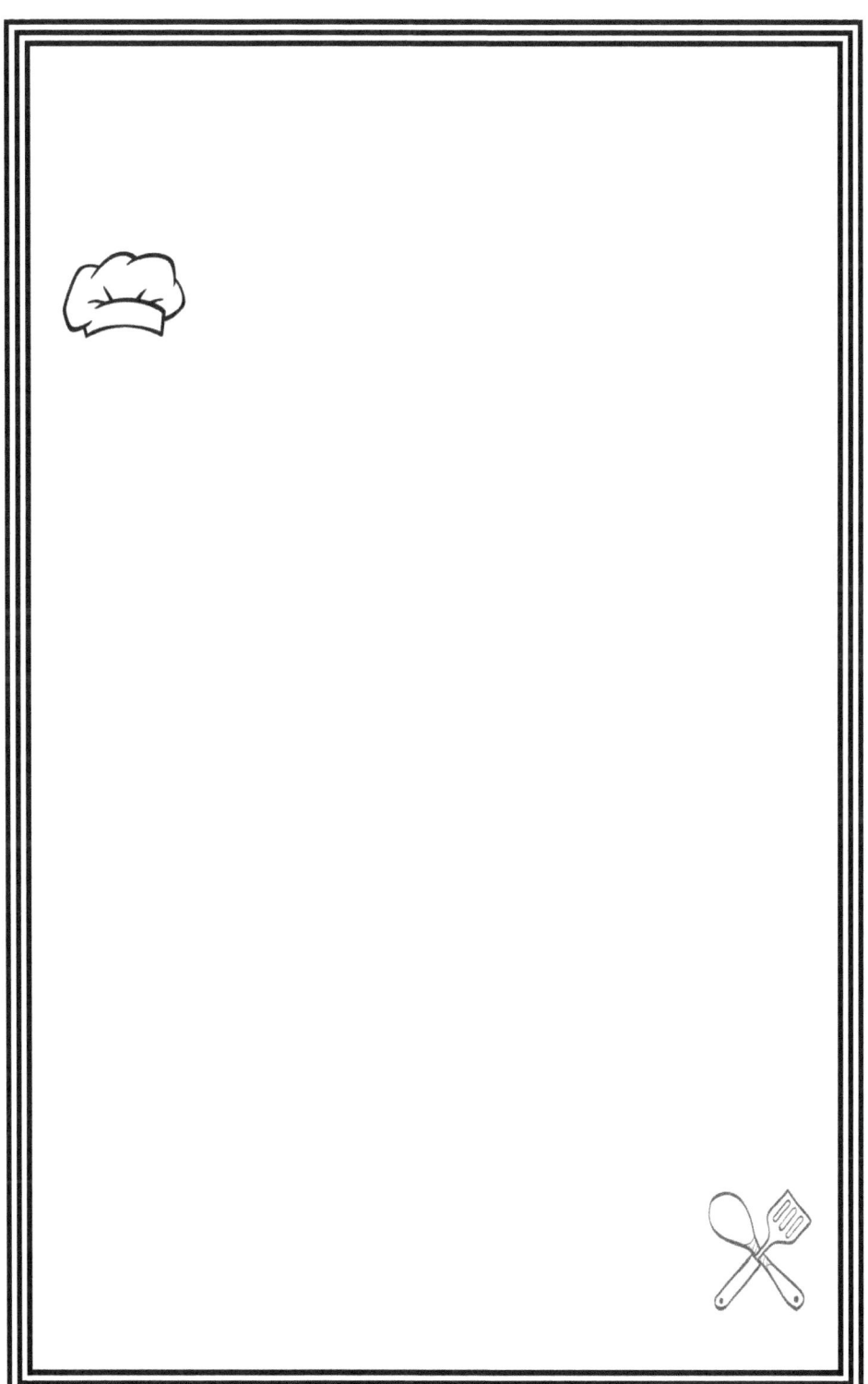

CHAPTER 2: MEAT RECIPES

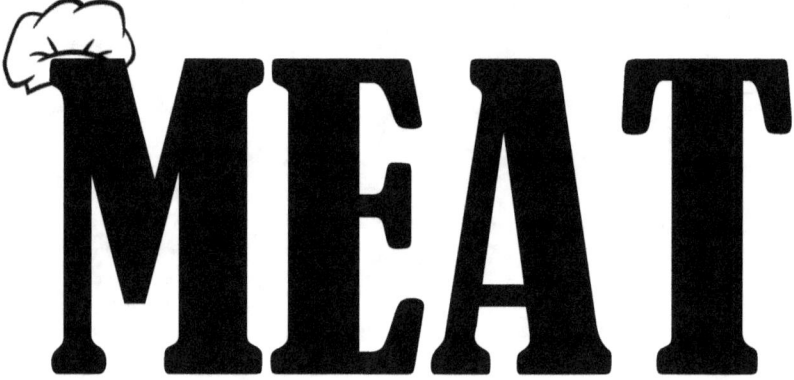

SAUSAGE BAKE

Prep:
15 mins
Cook:
1 hr 35 mins
Additional:
8 hrs
Total:
9 hrs 50 mins
Servings:
12
Yield:
12 servings

INGREDIENTS:

1 ½ pounds bulk pork sausage
3 ½ cups milk, divided
8 eggs
¾ teaspoon dry mustard
8 slices bread, torn into small squares
2 cups shredded mozzarella cheese
1 (10.75 ounce) can condensed cream of mushroom soup

DIRECTIONS:

1
Heat a large skillet over medium-high heat. Cook and stir sausage in the hot skillet until browned and crumbly, 5 to 7 minutes; drain and discard grease.

2
Beat 2 1/2 cups milk, eggs, and mustard in a large bowl.

3
Spread bread squares into the bottom of a baking dish. Layer mozzarella cheese atop the bread and top with sausage. Pour the egg mixture over the entire dish. Cover the baking dish with plastic wrap and refrigerate 8 hours to overnight.

4
Preheat oven to 300 degrees F (150 degrees C).

5
Stir cream of mushroom soup and 1 cup milk together in a bowl. Remove and discard plastic wrap from baking dish. Pour soup mixture over the 'bake.'

6
Bake in preheated oven until hot in the center, about 90 minutes.

NUTRITION FACTS:

342 calories; protein 20.5g; carbohydrates 14.7g; fat 22g; cholesterol 174.2mg;

STUFFED AND ROLLED PORK TENDERLOIN

Prep:
15 mins
Cook:
45 mins
Additional:
15 mins
Total:
1 hr 15 mins
Servings:
4

INGREDIENTS:

1 pork tenderloin
½ bunch flat-leaf parsley, chopped
⅓ cup bread crumbs
¼ cup dried currants
3 cloves garlic, minced
2 sprigs fresh rosemary, chopped
1 egg
2 tablespoons olive oil
2 teaspoons salt
1 ½ teaspoons ground black pepper
1 pinch cayenne pepper
salt and ground black pepper to taste

DIRECTIONS:

1
Preheat oven to 375 degrees F (190 degrees C).

2
Remove the flap of meat at the wider end of the tenderloin and trim the last two inches off of the narrow end of the tenderloin; chop trimmings and reserve.

3
Cut from one side of the tenderloin through the middle horizontally to within one-half inch of the other side. Open the two sides and spread them out like an open book. Cut a few shallow slashes in the meat. Cover the meat with plastic wrap and pound to about 1/2-inch thick. Roll up pounded tenderloin, cover with plastic wrap, and refrigerate to keep cold.

4
Mix chopped pork trimmings, parsley, bread crumbs, currants, garlic, rosemary, egg, olive oil, 2 teaspoons salt, 1 1/2 teaspoons black pepper, and cayenne pepper together in a bowl with a fork until stuffing is well-combined.

5
Unroll tenderloin on work surface. Spread stuffing over tenderloin, leaving a 2-inch border on one of the long-sides. Roll up tenderloin, ending at the 2-inch border; tie meat with twine to secure shape. Season tenderloin all over with salt and black pepper.

6
Heat an oven-safe skillet over high heat until hot. Cook tenderloin in hot skillet until browned, 3 to 4 minutes per side.

7

Cook in the preheated oven until pork is slightly pink in the center, about 30 minutes. An instant-read thermometer inserted into the center should read at least 145 degrees F (63 degrees C). Transfer to a plate and let rest for 15 minutes before removing twine and slicing.

NUTRITION FACTS:

284 calories; protein 23.7g; carbohydrates 15.1g; fat 14.1g; cholesterol 109.7mg; sodium 1294.9mg.

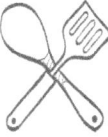

SWEET AND SOUR FAUX MEAT BALLS

Servings:
9
Yield:
8 to 10 servings

INGREDIENTS:

¼ cup vegetable oil
¼ cup distilled white vinegar
1 cup apricot jam
1 cup ketchup
¼ cup minced onion
1 teaspoon salt
1 teaspoon dried oregano
1 dash hot pepper sauce
5 eggs, beaten
1 cup shredded Cheddar cheese
½ cup cottage cheese
½ cup finely diced onion
1 cup chopped pecans
1 teaspoon dried basil
½ tablespoon salt
¼ teaspoon sage
2 cups Italian seasoned bread crumbs

DIRECTIONS:

1

To make Sweet and Sour Sauce: In a medium bowl combine the oil, vinegar, jam, ketchup, grated onion, salt, oregano and hot pepper sauce. Stir until well combined.

2

Preheat oven to 350 degrees F (175 degrees C).

3

In a large bowl combine the eggs, Cheddar cheese, cottage cheese, chopped onion, pecans, basil, salt, sage and bread crumbs. Mix well and form into 2 inch balls or patties. Place them in a 9x13 inch baking dish and cover them with sweet and sour sauce. Bake at 350 degrees F (175 degrees C) for 35 to 40 minutes.

NUTRITION FACTS:

462 calories; protein 14g; carbohydrates 51.7g; fat 24g; cholesterol 118.7mg;

CHEESEBURGER QUESADILLAS

Prep:
20 mins
Cook:
13 mins
Additional:
5 mins
Total:
38 mins
Servings:
4
Yield:
2 quesadillas

INGREDIENTS:

½ pound ground beef
½ red onion, diced
1 clove garlic, minced
1 pinch salt
1 cup shredded Cheddar cheese, divided
¼ cup shredded mozzarella cheese
1 tablespoon milk
1 tablespoon butter, divided
2 (12 inch) flour tortillas
2 tablespoons Thousand Island dressing, divided
1 romaine lettuce heart, sliced

1 tomato, sliced
½ red onion, sliced

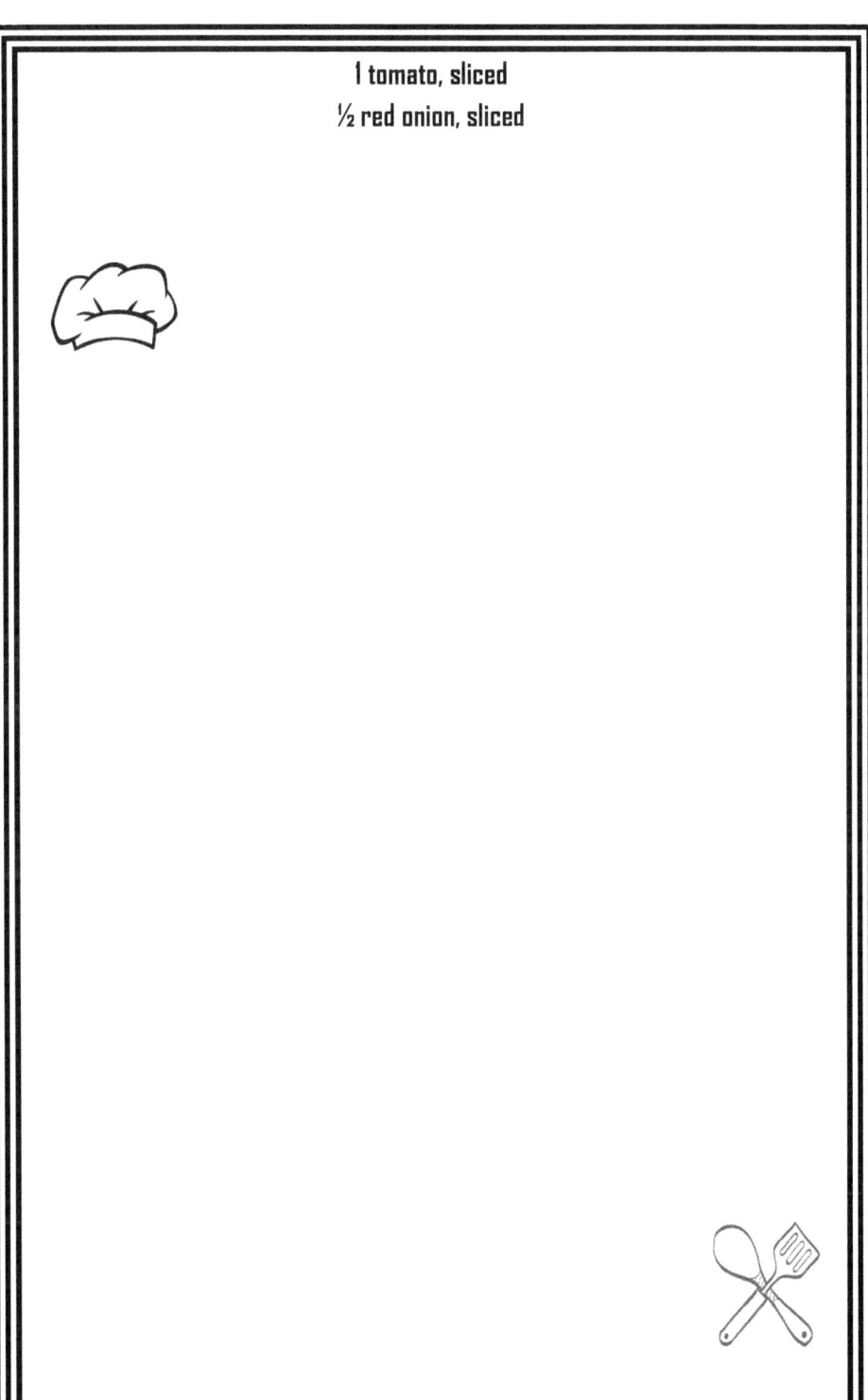

DIRECTIONS:

1

Combine beef, diced onion, and garlic in a large skillet; cook and stir until beef is no longer pink, 5 to 8 minutes. Season with salt.

2

Transfer beef to a saucepan over low heat. Add 3/4 cup Cheddar cheese, mozzarella cheese, and milk. Cook and stir until cheese is melted, 3 to 5 minutes.

3

Melt half the butter in a large skillet over medium heat. Cook 1 tortilla until golden brown on the bottom, about 3 minutes. Flip tortilla and spread with 1 tablespoon dressing. Spoon half of the beef mixture over the tortilla; fold in half. Cook until tortilla is golden brown, 1 to 2 minutes per side. Transfer to a serving plate. Repeat with second tortilla.

4

Sprinkle remaining 1/4 cup Cheddar cheese over tortillas. Let cool, about 5 minutes. Cut into wedges and serve with lettuce, tomato, and sliced onion.

NUTRITION FACTS:

521 calories; protein 24.4g; carbohydrates 38.4g; fat 30g; cholesterol 79.3mg; sodium 776.8mg

BEEF BULGOGI

Prep:
10 mins
Cook:
5 mins
Additional:
1 hr
Total:
1 hr 15 mins
Servings:
4
Yield:
4 servings

INGREDIENTS:

1 pound flank steak, thinly sliced
5 tablespoons soy sauce
2 ½ tablespoons white sugar
¼ cup chopped green onion
2 tablespoons minced garlic
2 tablespoons sesame seeds
2 tablespoons sesame oil
½ teaspoon ground black pepper

DIRECTIONS:

1
Place the beef in a shallow dish. Combine soy sauce, sugar, green onion, garlic, sesame seeds, sesame oil, and ground black pepper in a small bowl.
Pour over beef.
Cover and refrigerate for at least 1 hour or overnight.

2
Preheat an outdoor grill for high heat, and lightly oil the grate.

3
Quickly grill beef on hot grill until slightly charred and cooked through, 1 to 2 minutes per side.

NUTRITION FACTS:

232 calories; protein 16.2g; carbohydrates 12.4g; fat 13.2g; cholesterol 27.2mg;

PRESSURE COOKER CHUCK ROAST WITH VEGGIES AND GRAVY

Prep:
10 mins
Cook:
1 hr 15 mins
Additional:
15 mins
Total:
1 hr 40 mins
Servings:
12

INGREDIENTS:

1 (10 ounce) can condensed cream of celery soup
1 (1.5 ounce) package dry beef stew seasoning mix
1 (3 pound) boneless beef chuck roast
1 ½ cups beef broth
1 large yellow onion, quartered
1 (8 ounce) package sliced baby bella mushrooms (Optional)
1 pound baby red potatoes, halved
1 (16 ounce) package baby carrots

DIRECTIONS:

1

Mix celery soup and beef stew seasoning together in a small bowl to create a creamy paste.

2

Turn on a multi-functional pressure cooker and select Saute function. Add chuck roast and cook until juices start to render and outside is browned, about 5 minutes per side. Add the paste mixture, broth, onion, and mushrooms. Close and lock the lid. Select high pressure according to manufacturer's instructions; set timer for 40 minutes. Allow 10 to 15 minutes for pressure to build.

3

Release pressure carefully using the quick-release method according to manufacturer's instructions, about 5 minutes. Unlock and remove the lid. Add potatoes and carrots. Close, lock, and return cooker to high pressure. Cook for 15 minutes more.

4

Release pressure using the natural-release method according to manufacturer's instructions, 10 to 30 minutes. Transfer roast to a large bowl and shred with 2 forks; remove any excess fat. Run remaining liquid through a strainer into a separate bowl. Beat liquid with a whisk until well blended and emulsified, about 1 minute.

5

Serve shredded roast on top of the vegetables and cover with gravy.

NUTRITION FACTS:

250 calories; protein 15.5g; carbohydrates 14.7g; fat 14.1g; cholesterol 54.3mg;

BACON-WRAPPED DOUBLE DOGS

Prep:
15 mins
Cook:
10 mins
Total:
25 mins
Servings:
2
Yield:
2 servings

INGREDIENTS:

4 (2 ounce) hot dogs
4 slices cold center-cut, thinly sliced bacon
2 roll (blank)s large hot dog buns
2 tablespoons prepared yellow mustard, or to taste
2 tablespoons dill pickle relish, or to taste
2 teaspoons diced red onion, or to taste
2 tablespoons diced tomato, or to taste

DIRECTIONS:

1

Place 1 hot dog horizontally at the top edge of 1 bacon slice; roll once to secure. Place the second hot dog on the bacon, directly under the first hot dog, and wrap bacon twice at an angle.
Tuck between the hot dogs.
Tuck in second bacon slice where you left off and roll over remaining half of the hot dogs. Secure the end between the hot dogs. Repeat with remaining hot dogs and bacon slices.

2

Heat a nonstick pan over medium heat and add bacon-wrapped hot dogs. Cook, turning as needed, until browned on all sides, about 10 minutes.

3

Spread 1 tablespoon mustard over each bun. Add hot dogs. Top with dill pickle relish, red onion, and tomato.

NUTRITION FACTS:

607 calories; protein 24.4g; carbohydrates 28g; fat 43.6g; cholesterol 79.9mg;

SESAME SAKE PORK MEDALLIONS

Prep:
30 mins
Total:
30 mins
Servings:
4
Yield:
4 servings

INGREDIENTS:

1 cup Cooking Wine
2 tablespoons brown sugar, not packed
1 teaspoon toasted sesame oil
1 teaspoon cornstarch
1 ½ pounds pork tenderloin
2 tablespoons toasted sesame seeds, or more if desired
2 tablespoons butter
Minced green onion (garnish)

DIRECTIONS:

1

Combine sake cooking wine, sugar, sesame oil and cornstarch. Stir to dissolve cornstarch; set aside.

2

Cut pork into 1/2-inch slices; season with salt and pepper to taste. Press half the sesame seeds onto one side of each medallion. Melt butter in 12-inch saute pan. Cook pork, seed side down, over medium-high heat until lightly browned, about 8 minutes. While cooking, press remaining sesame seeds onto tops of medallions. Turn over and continue to cook 4-6 minutes. Increase heat to high, add sauce and cook 2 minutes or until sauce bubbles and thickens slightly. Serve pork medallions drizzled with sake sauce. Sprinkle with any remaining sesame seeds and green onion.

NUTRITION FACTS:

359 calories; protein 31g; carbohydrates 10.4g; fat 17.4g; cholesterol 110mg; sodium 488.1mg.

BALSAMIC ROASTED BRUSSELS SPROUTS WITH BACON

Prep:
15 mins
Cook:
15 mins
Total:
30 mins
Servings:
4
Yield:
4 servings

INGREDIENTS:

1 pound Brussels sprouts, trimmed and halved or quartered
2 tablespoons balsamic vinegar, divided
1 tablespoon olive oil
¼ teaspoon salt
¼ teaspoon ground black pepper
2 slices bacon
2 teaspoons lemon zest (Optional)

DIRECTIONS:

1

Preheat the oven to 400 degrees F (200 degrees C). Line a 15x10-inch baking pan with foil.

2

Place Brussels sprouts into the prepared pan. Drizzle with 1 tablespoon balsamic vinegar and olive oil. Season with salt and pepper; toss to coat.

3

Roast in the preheated oven until Brussels sprouts are crisp-tender and brown, stirring every 5 minutes, 15 to 20 minutes total.

4

While the Brussels sprouts are roasting, place bacon in a large skillet and cook over medium-high heat, turning occasionally, until evenly browned and crisp, 10 to 12 minutes. Drain bacon slices on paper towels. Crumble when cool enough to handle.

5

Drizzle roasted Brussels sprouts with remaining 1 tablespoon balsamic vinegar and sprinkle with crumbled bacon and lemon zest.

NUTRITION FACTS:

93 calories; protein 4.4g; carbohydrates 11.6g; fat 4.5g; cholesterol 1.9mg; sodium 212.1mg.

ITALIAN MINI MEAT LOAVES

Prep:
10 mins
Cook:
45 mins
Total:
55 mins
Servings:
4
Yield:
4 mini meat loaves

INGREDIENTS:

2 tablespoons olive oil
1 pound lean ground beef
8 ounces bulk mild Italian sausage
½ cup diced white onion
1 (24 ounce) jar Classico® Fresh Four Cheese Sauce, divided
1 egg, lightly beaten
⅓ cup Italian seasoned bread crumbs
¼ cup shredded Parmesan cheese
¼ teaspoon garlic powder
½ teaspoon salt
⅛ teaspoon black pepper
1 tablespoon chopped fresh parsley
1 cup shredded mozzarella cheese

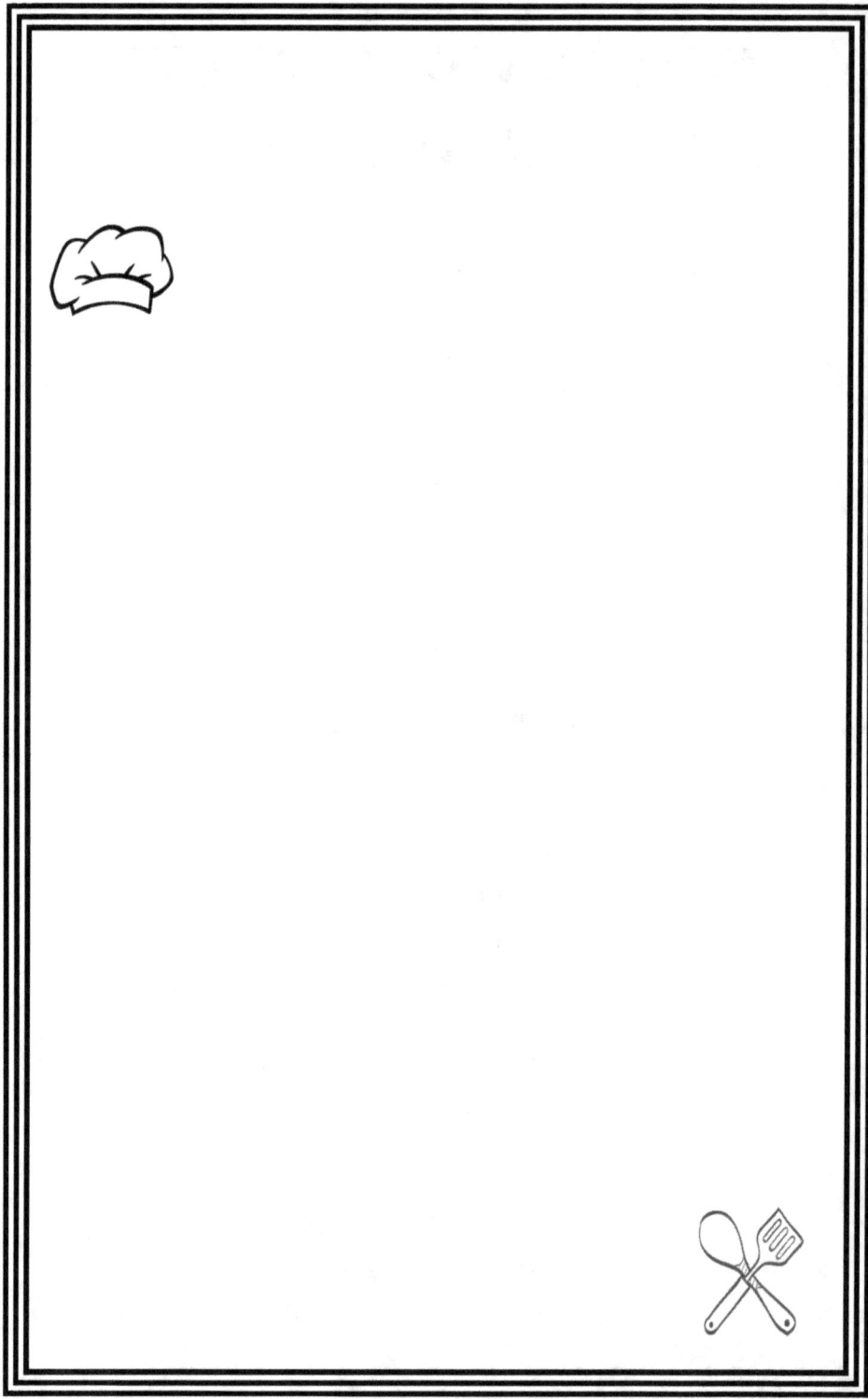

DIRECTIONS:

1

Heat oven to 350 degrees F. Generously oil the bottom of a 9x13-inch baking dish.

2

Mix together the ground beef and Italian sausage in a large bowl. Add onion, half of the jar of four-cheese red sauce, egg, bread crumbs, Parmesan cheese, garlic powder, salt, pepper, and parsley. Mix until well blended.

3

Divide mixture into 4 oval mini loaves; place in prepared baking dish. Pour the remaining red sauce over tops of meat loaves.

4

Spray the underside of a large piece of foil with nonstick cooking spray; cover dish tightly.

5

Bake for 45 minutes. Uncover and sprinkle loaves with shredded mozzarella cheese.

6

Increase the oven temperature to 400 degrees F. Bake uncovered until cheese is melted and the internal temperature reaches 165 degrees F, about 10 more minutes.

NUTRITION FACTS:

675 calories; protein 43.6g; carbohydrates 27.8g; fat 42.9g; cholesterol 172.1mg;

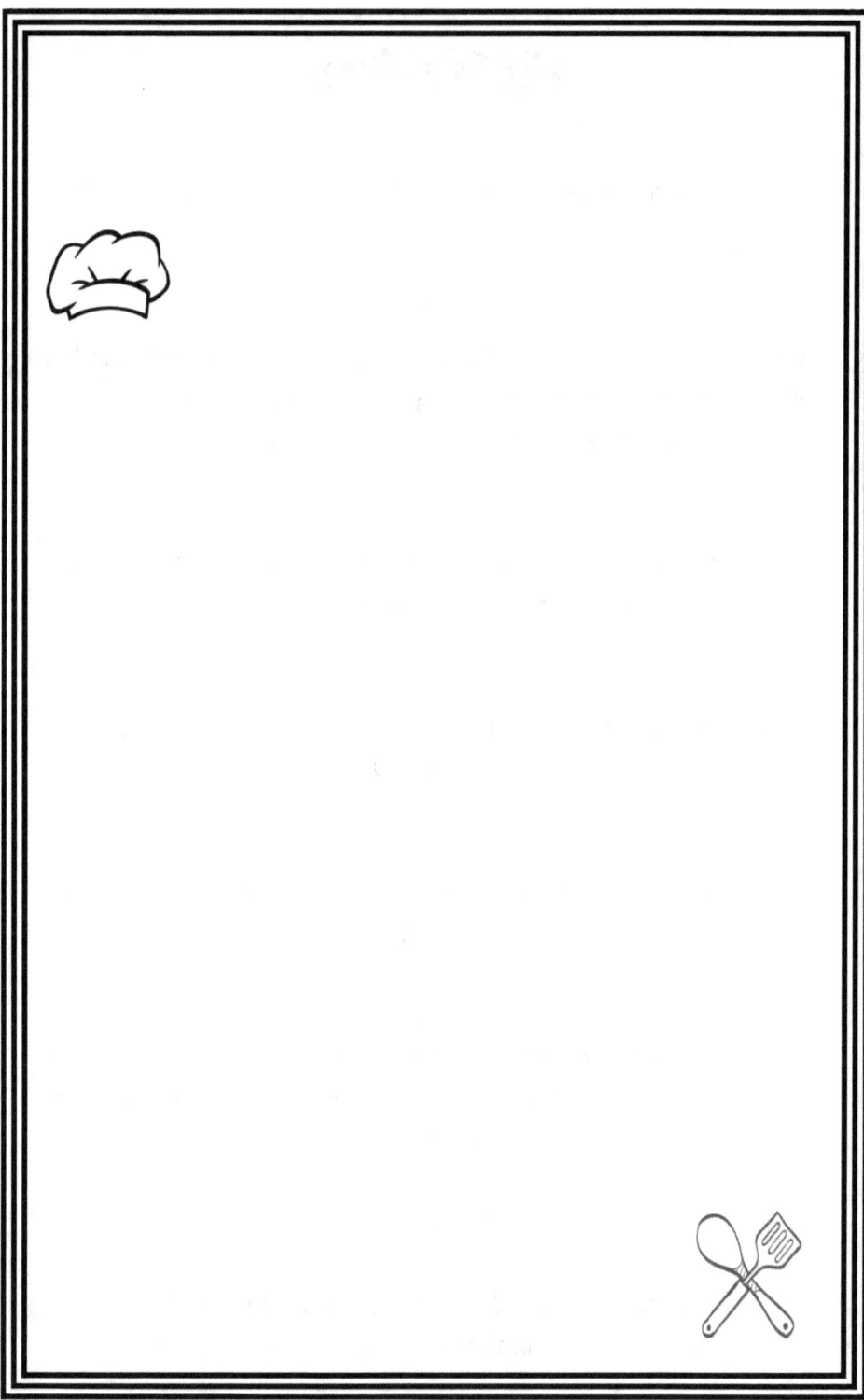

CHAPTER 3: FISH & SEAFOOD RECIPES

BELL PEPPER AND LEMON SALMON

Prep:
15 mins
Cook:
35 mins
Additional:
1 hr
Total:
1 hr 50 mins
Servings:
2
Yield:
2 servings

INGREDIENTS:

¼ cup olive oil
2 cloves garlic, chopped
1 lemon, juiced
1 pinch kosher salt
2 (8 ounce) salmon fillets
2 tablespoons capers, drained and rinsed
½ red bell pepper, cut into 1/4-inch strips

DIRECTIONS:

1

In a shallow dish, mix the olive oil, garlic, lemon juice, and salt. Pierce the salmon fillets on both sides with a fork, and place in the dish. Coat with the olive oil mixture, and marinate at least 1 hour in the refrigerator.

2

Preheat oven to 375 degrees F (190 degrees C).

3

Place each salmon fillet on a large sheet of aluminum foil. Fold the foil around the fillets to form packets. Pour the marinade mixture over the fillets, and top with capers and red bell pepper strips. Tightly seal packets, and place in a baking dish.

4

Cook salmon 35 minutes in the preheated oven, until easily flaked with a fork.

NUTRITION FACTS:

627 calories; protein 40.1g; carbohydrates 9g; fat 49g; cholesterol 110.6mg;

BAKED HADDOCK

Prep:
10 mins
Cook:
15 mins
Total:
25 mins
Servings:
4
Yield:
4 servings

INGREDIENTS:

¾ cup milk
2 teaspoons salt
¾ cup bread crumbs
¼ cup grated Parmesan cheese
¼ teaspoon ground dried thyme
4 haddock fillets
¼ cup butter, melted

DIRECTIONS:

1

Preheat oven to 500 degrees F (260 degrees C).

2

In a small bowl, combine the milk and salt.
In a separate bowl, mix together the bread crumbs, Parmesan cheese, and thyme. Dip the haddock fillets in the milk, then press into the crumb mixture to coat. Place haddock fillets in a glass baking dish, and drizzle with melted butter.

3

Bake on the top rack of the preheated oven until the fish flakes easily, about 15 minutes.

NUTRITION FACTS:

325 calories; protein 27.7g; carbohydrates 17g; fat 15.7g; cholesterol 103.3mg;

SHRIMP AND VEGGIE STUFFED ZUCCHINI

Prep:
20 mins
Cook:
35 mins
Total:
55 mins
Servings:
4
Yield:
4 servings

INGREDIENTS:

1 extra large zucchini
¼ cup olive oil, divided
6 cloves garlic, finely chopped
1 shallot, finely chopped
½ pound large shrimp - shelled, deveined, and cut in half
1 large tomato - peeled, seeded and diced
8 cremini mushrooms, quartered
¼ cup grated Parmesan cheese
8 leaves fresh basil, torn
ground black pepper to taste
kosher salt to taste
garlic powder to taste
¼ cup grated Parmesan cheese, divided

DIRECTIONS:

1

Preheat the oven's broiler and set the oven rack about 6 inches from the heat source. Grease a baking sheet.

2

Cut the zucchini in half the long way, and scoop out the seeds and pulp, leaving a thick shell of flesh. Brush both halves of the zucchini with about 1 tablespoon of olive oil, and place them, cut sides down, onto the prepared baking sheet. Bake until the zucchini are hot and beginning to release beads of moisture, 5 to 10 minutes. Remove the zucchini from the oven.

3

Reduce the oven heat to 450 degrees F (230 degrees C).

4

Heat 2 tablespoons of olive oil in a skillet over medium-low heat, and cook and stir the garlic and shallot until translucent, about 5 minutes. Remove from the heat and let cool.

5

Place 1 tablespoon of olive oil, the shrimp, diced tomato, mushrooms, 1/4 cup of Parmesan cheese, basil, and the cooked garlic and shallot into a bowl, and stir to mix. Season to taste with black pepper, salt, and garlic powder. Stuff the mixture into the zucchini halves, and sprinkle each zucchini with about 2 tablespoons of Parmesan cheese.

6

Bake the stuffed zucchini in the preheated oven until the cheese is browned and the filling is cooked through and hot, about 20 minutes.

NUTRITION FACTS:

267 calories; protein 17.4g; carbohydrates 13g; fat 17.4g; cholesterol 95.1mg; sodium 375.8mg.

CHAPTER 4:

VEGETABLE

RECIPES

EGGPLANT GRATIN

Prep:
15 mins
Cook:
45 mins
Additional:
20 mins
Total:
1 hr 20 mins
Servings:
4
Yield:
4 servings

INGREDIENTS:

4 eggplants
salt and freshly ground black pepper to taste
1 (8 ounce) package feta cheese
1 cup heavy whipping cream
3 cloves garlic, minced
1 tablespoon chopped fresh parsley, or more to taste
1 tablespoon chopped fresh basil, or more to taste
1 splash olive oil
4 ripe tomatoes, sliced
2 yellow bell peppers, chopped

DIRECTIONS:

1

Slice eggplants in such a way that the slices are still connected at the bottom. Sprinkle with salt and set aside for 20 minutes. Wash off salt under running cold water and pat dry.

2

Preheat oven to 400 degrees F (200 degrees C). Grease a baking dish.

3

Mash feta cheese and cream together with a fork. Mix in garlic, parsley, basil, olive oil, salt, and pepper.

4

Place eggplants with the cut-side up into the prepared baking dish. Arrange tomato slices and bell pepper pieces alternately in between the eggplant slices. Pour feta-mixture over eggplants and cover with aluminum foil.

5

Bake in the preheated oven until feta cheese is melted and eggplants are cooked through, about 45 minutes. Sprinkle with more parsley.

NUTRITION FACTS:

549 calories; protein 17g; carbohydrates 46.7g; fat 36.8g; cholesterol 132mg;

GRILLED BROCCOLI RABE

Prep:
15 mins
Cook:
10 mins
Total:
25 mins
Servings:
4
Yield:
4 servings

INGREDIENTS:

1 bunch broccoli rabe, trimmed and rinsed
1 tablespoon olive oil
1 tablespoon lemon juice
¼ teaspoon crushed red pepper flakes
salt to taste

DIRECTIONS:

1

Bring a large pot of salted water to a boil. Set up an ice bath nearby. Place half of the broccoli rabe into the boiling water and cook for 1 minute, then remove with tongs to the ice bath to stop cooking. Repeat with remaining broccoli rabe. Place broccoli rabe into a large colander to drain.

2

Preheat an outdoor grill for medium-low heat, and lightly oil grate.

3

Whisk together olive oil, lemon juice, crushed red pepper flakes, and salt in a small bowl. Toss drained broccoli rabe with oil mixture, then place onto hot grate.

4

Grill, turning occasionally, until thick stems have softened, 8 to 10 minutes. Remove thinner leafy pieces as they become done to prevent burning. Remove to a serving platter.

NUTRITION FACTS:

8 calories; protein 2g; carbohydrates 3.1g; fat 3.4g; sodium 55.6mg.

BAKED MASHED PARSNIPS

Prep:
15 mins
Cook:
45 mins
Total:
1 hr
Servings:
6
Yield:
6 servings

INGREDIENTS:

3 pounds parsnips, peeled and cut into 1/2-inch pieces
¼ pound butter, melted
¼ cup sherry
¼ cup heavy whipping cream
1 teaspoon salt
1 teaspoon white sugar
¼ cup bread crumbs, or to taste
2 tablespoons butter, cut into small pieces, or more to taste

DIRECTIONS:

1
Place parsnips into a large pot and cover with water; bring to a boil. Reduce heat to medium-low and simmer until tender, 20 to 30 minutes. Drain and cool slightly.

2
Preheat oven to 350 degrees F (175 degrees C).

3
Beat parsnips, melted butter, sherry, heavy whipping cream, salt, and white sugar together in a bowl until smooth. Spoon into a baking dish and top with bread crumbs; dot with butter pieces.

4
Bake in the preheated oven until golden, 25 to 30 minutes.

NUTRITION FACTS:

401 calories; protein 3.7g; carbohydrates 45.9g; fat 23.8g; cholesterol 64.4mg;

ROASTED VEGETABLES WITH SPAGHETTI SQUASH

Prep:
15 mins
Cook:
1 hr 30 mins
Total:
1 hr 45 mins
Servings:
8
Yield:
8 servings

INGREDIENTS:

cooking spray
1 large spaghetti squash, halved and seeded
1 acorn squash, halved and seeded
1 large sweet potato
3 cups baby carrots
1 onion, diced
¼ cup honey
1 teaspoon ground cinnamon
1 pinch salt
1 pinch ground black pepper
⅓ cup shredded Cheddar cheese

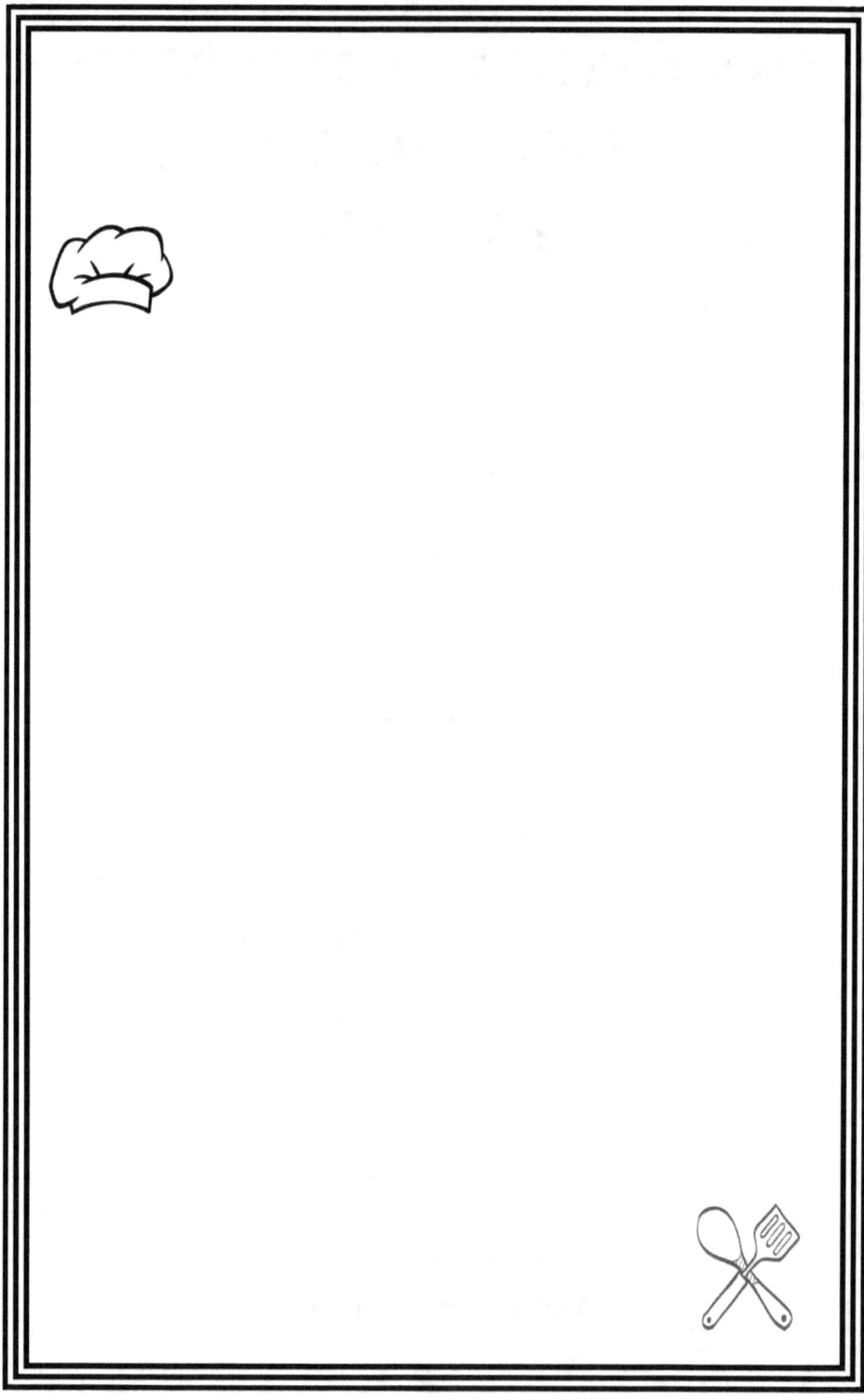

DIRECTIONS:

1

Preheat oven to 400 degrees F (205 degrees C). Coat a large baking sheet with cooking spray.

2

Place spaghetti squash and acorn squash, cut sides down, on baking sheet. Place sweet potato on baking sheet.

3

Bake until squash and sweet potato are tender when pierced by a fork, about 45 minutes.

4

Turn oven down to 350 degrees (170 degrees C). Coat a 9x13 baking dish with cooking spray.

5

Scrape strands from the spaghetti squash and place into prepared pan in an even layer.

6

Cut sweet potato into bite-size chunks; place into a large bowl. Scoop bite-size chunks of flesh from the acorn squash; add to bowl. Stir baby carrots, diced onion, honey, cinnamon, salt, and black pepper into squash mixture and mix well. Transfer squash mixture to the baking pan and spread evenly over spaghetti squash. Sprinkle Cheddar cheese over the top.

7

Bake at 350 degrees until cheese is bubbly and brown, about 45 minutes.

NUTRITION FACTS:

230 calories; protein 5g; carbohydrates 49.5g; fat 3.4g; cholesterol 6mg; sodium 148.2mg

HALLOUMI PARMIGIANA

Prep:
30 mins
Cook:
30 mins
Total:
1 hr
Servings:
4
Yield:
4 servings

INGREDIENTS:

1 small eggplant, cut into 1/2-inch rounds
1 tablespoon salt
1 large egg
1 cup bread crumbs
2 teaspoons dried oregano
½ teaspoon ground black pepper
¼ teaspoon ground cayenne pepper
1 cup oil for frying, or as needed
1 (8.8 ounce) package halloumi cheese, cut into 4 sticks
½ (16 ounce) package spaghetti
1 tablespoon extra-virgin olive oil
1 ¼ cups spaghetti sauce
8 tablespoons finely grated Parmigiano-Reggiano cheese

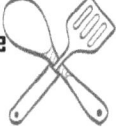

DIRECTIONS:

1

Place sliced eggplant into a large pot. Cover with salt and add enough water to cover. Place a plate on top of the rounds to keep them submerged; allow to sit for 10 minutes.

2

While eggplant soaks, whisk egg in a shallow dish. Combine bread crumbs, oregano, black pepper, and cayenne pepper in another shallow dish.

3

Heat oil in a deep skillet over medium-high heat.

4

Drain eggplant and discard water. Rinse eggplant and squeeze out as much water as possible. Pat slices dry with paper towels. Dredge eggplant slices in egg and then bread crumb mixture and place on a plate. Dredge halloumi cheese sticks in egg and then bread crumb mixture and place on a plate.

5

Fry breaded eggplant slices in the hot oil until browned, about 2 minutes. Flip and fry on the other side, about 2 minutes more. Drain on clean paper towels. Repeat with halloumi cheese sticks.

6

Meanwhile bring a large pot of lightly salted water to a boil. Cook spaghetti in the boiling water, stirring occasionally, until tender yet firm to the bite, about 12 minutes. Toss cooked pasta with extra-virgin olive oil.

7
Pour spaghetti sauce into a small saucepan and heat over medium heat until hot, about 5 minutes.

8
Divide cooked spaghetti onto 4 plates. Evenly distribute eggplant and halloumi cheese. Top with equal amounts of spaghetti sauce and Parmigiano-Reggiano cheese.

NUTRITION FACTS:

1179 calories; protein 32g; carbohydrates 79.6g; fat 82.7g

HABANERO COOKIES

Prep:
25 mins
Cook:
10 mins
Additional:
10 mins
Total:
45 mins
Servings:
24
Yield:
2 dozen cookies

INGREDIENTS:

10 habanero peppers, seeded and minced
1 ½ cups white sugar
1 cup softened butter
1 teaspoon vanilla extract
2 eggs
2 ¾ cups all-purpose flour
1 teaspoon baking soda
1 teaspoon salt

DIRECTIONS:

1
Preheat oven to 325 degrees F (165 degrees C).

2
In a large bowl, mix the peppers, sugar, butter, vanilla, and eggs. Beat until smooth. In a separate bowl, sift together the flour, baking soda, and salt. Stir into the pepper mixture just until combined. Drop by rounded teaspoonfuls onto ungreased cookie sheets.

3
Bake 10 minutes in the preheated oven, or until golden brown. Cool on wire racks.

NUTRITION FACTS:

176 calories; protein 2.1g; carbohydrates 23.7g; fat 8.2g; cholesterol 35.8mg; sodium 210.2mg.

VEGETARIAN SPINACH AND MUSHROOM ENCHILADAS

Prep:
30 mins
Cook:
35 mins
Total:
1 hr 5 mins
Servings:
10
Yield:
10 servings

INGREDIENTS:

3 tablespoons butter
1 pound mushrooms, cleaned and sliced
1 cup coarsely chopped onion
8 ounces fresh spinach - washed, stemmed, and coarsely chopped
salt and ground black pepper to taste
1 (10 ounce) can Mexican-style diced tomatoes with lime and cilantro (such as Rotel®), half drained
1 (8 ounce) package neufchatel cheese
1 (16 ounce) container sour cream, divided
½ teaspoon ground cumin
20 corn tortillas

1 pound shredded Monterey Jack cheese
1 (8 ounce) jar salsa, or as needed

DIRECTIONS:

1

Preheat the oven to 350 degrees F (175 degrees C). Lightly grease a 9x13-inch baking dish.

2

Heat a skillet over high heat. Add butter, mushrooms, and onion and cook until onions are translucent, 7 to 10 minutes. Add spinach and toss until wilted, about 3 minutes more. Season with salt and pepper. Remove from heat and set aside.

3

Heat a small saucepan over medium heat. Add diced tomatoes, neufchatel cheese, 8 ounces sour cream, and cumin. Stir until thoroughly mixed, about 1 minute, and remove from heat.

4

Place tortillas between 2 paper towels and heat in a microwave oven until warm, 30 seconds to 1 minute.

5

Scoop about 2 tablespoons spinach mixture, 1 tablespoon cream mixture, and 1 to 2 tablespoons shredded Monterey Jack cheese into a tortilla. Roll up and place seam-side down in the prepared baking dish. Repeat with remaining tortillas. Spread any remaining cream mixture on top of enchiladas. Sprinkle any remaining Monterey Jack cheese on top. Cover.

6

Bake in the preheated oven until heated through, about 20 minutes.

7
Garnish individual servings with remaining sour cream and salsa.

NUTRITION FACTS:

501 calories; protein 20.6g; carbohydrates 32.4g; fat 33.8g; cholesterol 86.6mg; sodium 687.7mg

VEGAN BLUEBERRY MUFFINS

Prep:
15 mins
Cook:
18 mins
Additional:
5 mins
Total:
38 mins
Servings:
12
Yield:
12 muffins

INGREDIENTS:

2 cups all-purpose flour
2 ½ teaspoons baking powder
½ teaspoon baking soda
½ teaspoon salt
½ cup white sugar
2 tablespoons white sugar
½ cup unsweetened applesauce
½ cup vanilla soy yogurt
¼ cup vegetable oil
2 teaspoons vanilla sugar
1 teaspoon vanilla extract

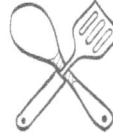

1 ¾ cups fresh blueberries
2 tablespoons brown sugar

DIRECTIONS:

tep 1
Preheat oven to 350 degrees F (175 degrees C). Grease a 12-cup muffin tin or line cups with paper liners.

2
Combine flour, baking powder, baking soda, and salt in a large bowl. Stir together 1/2 cup plus 2 tablespoons white sugar, unsweetened applesauce, yogurt, oil, vanilla sugar, and vanilla extract in a second bowl. Fold into flour mixture using a spatula, but do not over mix. Fold in blueberries.

3
Spoon batter into the prepared muffin cups, filling each 3/4 full. Sprinkle with brown sugar.

4
Bake in the preheated oven until tops spring back when lightly pressed, 18 to 22 minutes. Cool in the tin for 5 minutes. Transfer to a wire rack to cool completely.

NUTRITION FACTS:

193 calories; protein 2.9g; carbohydrates 34.2g; fat 5.3g; sodium 253.2mg.

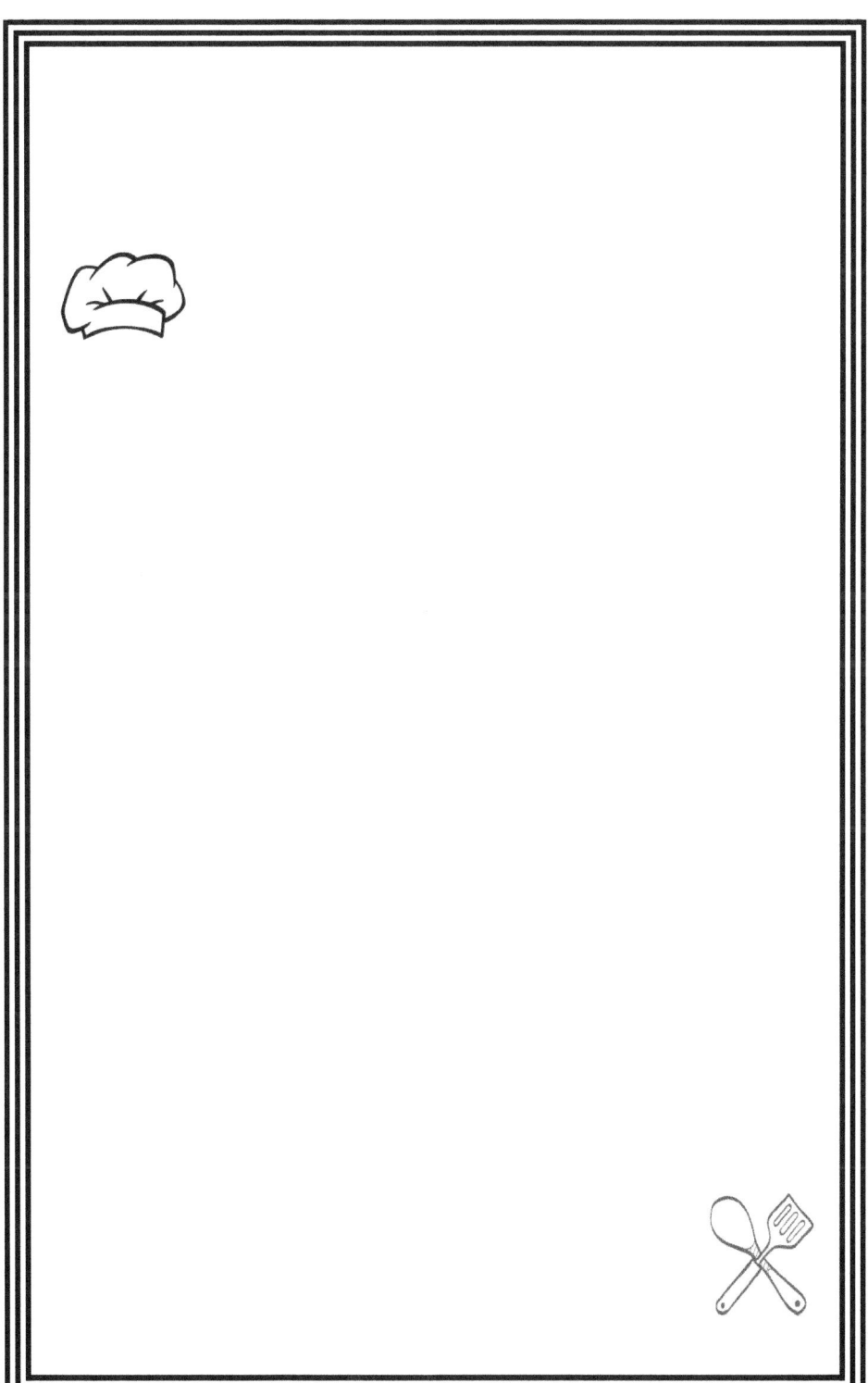

CHAPTER 5: SNACK & APPETIZERS RECIPES

BACON WRAPPED STUFFED MUSHROOMS

Prep:
10 mins
Cook:
20 mins
Total:
30 mins
Servings:
20
Yield:
20 appetizers

INGREDIENTS:

½ cup chopped green onions
2 (8 ounce) packages cream cheese, softened
20 fresh mushrooms, stems removed
1 pound sliced bacon, cut in half

DIRECTIONS:

1

Preheat the oven to 350 degrees F (175 degrees C).

2

In a medium bowl, mix together
the green onions and cream cheese .
Stuff mushroom caps with the cheese mixture.
Wrap each mushroom with a half-slice of bacon, and secure with toothpicks.
Place on a baking sheet.

3

Bake for 20 minutes in the preheated oven, until the bacon is cooked through.

NUTRITION FACTS:

123 calories; protein 5.1g; carbohydrates 1.5g; fat 11g; cholesterol 32.8mg;

BAKED WALNUTS

Prep:
10 mins
Cook:
30 mins
Total:
40 mins
Servings:
16
Yield:
1 pound

INGREDIENTS:

2 egg whites, stiffly beaten
1 cup white sugar
½ cup butter, softened
1 pound walnut halves

DIRECTIONS:

1
Preheat oven to 350 degrees F (175 degrees C).

2
To the stiff egg whites add sugar, butter and walnuts. Mix until nuts are well coated. Spread out on a cookie sheet.

3
Bake in preheated oven for 20 to 30 minutes, stirring a couple of times, until browned.

NUTRITION FACTS:

287 calories; protein 4.8g; carbohydrates 16.4g; fat 24.3g; cholesterol 15.3mg; sodium 48.4mg.

BACON-WRAPPED MEATLOAF

Prep:
25 mins
Cook:
1 hr 30 mins
Additional:
5 mins
Total:
2 hrs
Servings:
6
Yield:
1 meatloaf

INGREDIENTS:

1 pound ground beef
½ pound ground pork sausage
1 sleeve crushed buttery round crackers (such as Ritz®)
⅔ cup ketchup
½ cup chopped onion
2 eggs
1 teaspoon onion powder
1 teaspoon garlic powder
12 slices thick-cut bacon

DIRECTIONS:

1

Preheat the oven to 350 degrees F (175 degrees C).

2

Combine ground beef, ground sausage, crushed crackers, ketchup, onion, eggs, onion powder, and garlic powder in a large bowl until mixed thoroughly, using your hands for best results. Form mixture into a loaf shape.

3

Weave strips of bacon into a basket weave pattern. Place meatloaf in the center and carefully lift and transfer to a loaf pan, so bacon is on the bottom and sides of the pan.

4

Bake in the preheated oven until no longer pink in the center, about 1 1/2 hours. An instant-read thermometer inserted into the center should read at least 165 degrees F (74 degrees C). Allow to sit for 5 minutes before carefully flipping onto a platter.

NUTRITION FACTS:

403 calories; protein 26.7g; carbohydrates 9.2g; fat 28.4g; cholesterol 149.1mg;

TURNIP BAKE

Prep:
20 mins
Cook:
1 hr 15 mins
Total:
1 hr 35 mins
Servings:
8
Yield:
8 servings

INGREDIENTS:

1 large turnip, peeled and cubed
2 tablespoons butter
1 pinch salt and ground black pepper
2 large apples - peeled, cored, and diced
2 tablespoons brown sugar
1 pinch ground cinnamon

Topping:

¼ cup all-purpose flour
¼ cup brown sugar
2 tablespoons butter, softened

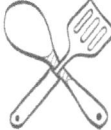

DIRECTIONS:

1

Preheat oven to 350 degrees F (175 degrees C). Grease an 8-inch casserole dish.

2

Place turnip into a large pot and cover with salted water; bring to a boil. Reduce heat to medium-low and simmer until tender, 15 to 20 minutes. Drain and transfer to a bowl.

3

Mash turnip, 2 tablespoons butter, salt, and pepper together until smooth.

4

Toss apples with 2 tablespoons brown sugar and cinnamon in a bowl.

5

Spread half the turnip mixture into the prepared casserole dish; top with half the apples. Repeat with remaining turnip mixture and apple mixture.

6

Mix flour, 1/4 cup brown sugar, and 2 tablespoons softened butter by hand in a bowl until mixture is an evenly coarse meal-texture; sprinkle over casserole.

7

Bake in the preheated oven until cooked through and bubbling, about 1 hour.

NUTRITION FACTS:

138 calories; protein 0.8g; carbohydrates 21.9g; fat 5.9g;

SAUSAGE-STUFFED PIQUILLO PEPPERS

Prep:
15 mins
Cook:
20 mins
Additional:
10 mins
Total:
45 mins

INGREDIENTS:

8 teaspoons olive oil, or as needed, divided
4 ounces chorizo sausage, casings removed and meat crumbled
½ cup diced green onion
salt and ground black pepper to taste
½ cup cooked long-grain white rice
2 ounces goat cheese
1 large egg
3 tablespoons chopped fresh parsley, divided
2 cloves garlic, crushed
1 teaspoon ground cumin
1 blood orange, zested and juiced
1 pinch cayenne pepper, or more to taste
12 piquillo peppers
2 tablespoons chopped almonds

DIRECTIONS:

1

Preheat oven to 400 degrees F (200 degrees C). Brush a baking dish with 1 tablespoon olive oil.

2

Heat 1 tablespoon olive oil in a skillet over medium-high heat. Saute sausage, green onion, and a pinch of salt in hot oil until meat is browned and crumbly and onion is translucent, 5 to 7 minutes. Remove from heat and cool for 10 minutes.

3

Mix rice, goat cheese, egg, 2 tablespoons parsley, garlic, cumin, 1 teaspoon blood orange zest, and cayenne pepper together in a bowl. Spoon rice mixture into each pepper. Place stuffed peppers in a single layer in the prepared baking dish. Scatter almonds over the top, drizzle with 1 teaspoon olive oil, and sprinkle with salt.

4

Bake in the preheated oven until stuffed peppers are heated through and filling is hot, 15 to 20 minutes. Drizzle 1 tablespoon blood orange juice, remaining 1 teaspoon olive oil, and remaining parsley over the top.

NUTRITION FACTS:

128 calories; protein 5g; carbohydrates 6.8g; fat 9.4g; cholesterol 27.5mg;

ROASTED GREEN BEANS AND SHALLOTS

Prep:
15 mins
Cook:
10 mins
Total:
25 mins
Servings:
6
Yield:
6 servings

INGREDIENTS:

1 ½ pounds fresh green beans, trimmed
6 shallots, peeled and thinly sliced
5 large cloves garlic, thinly sliced
¼ cup sliced almonds
2 tablespoons olive oil, or more as needed
1 teaspoon kosher salt
½ teaspoon freshly ground black pepper

DIRECTIONS:

1

Preheat the oven to 425 degrees F (220 degrees C). Line a baking sheet with parchment paper.

2

Place green beans in a large bowl. Mix in shallots, garlic, and almonds. Drizzle olive oil over the top; sprinkle salt and pepper evenly on top. Toss until everything is evenly coated with oil. Spread in a single layer on the prepared baking sheet.

3

Roast in the preheated oven until beans are slightly shriveled and shallots are lightly browned, 10 to 15 minutes.

NUTRITION FACTS:

141 calories; protein 4.4g; carbohydrates 18.7g; fat 6.7g; sodium 333.7mg.

ROASTED RADISHES WITH ONIONS

Prep:
15 mins
Cook:
20 mins
Total:
35 mins
Servings:
4
Yield:
4 servings

INGREDIENTS:

1 bunch radishes, trimmed and halved
1 medium onion, halved and sliced
½ teaspoon lemon zest
¼ teaspoon dried thyme
¼ teaspoon dried dill
¼ teaspoon garlic powder
1 pinch salt and ground black pepper to taste
3 tablespoons olive oil

DIRECTIONS:

1

Preheat the oven to 400 degrees F (200 degrees C). Line a baking sheet with parchment paper.

2

Place radishes and onion in a medium bowl. Sprinkle with lemon zest, thyme, dill, garlic powder, salt, and pepper. Drizzle with olive oil and toss to coat. Spread on the baking sheet in an even layer.

3

Roast in the preheated oven, stirring every 5 to 10 minutes, until edges are beginning to brown and radishes are fork-tender, 20 to 25 minutes. Taste and season with additional salt, if desired.

NUTRITION FACTS:

105 calories; protein 0.5g; carbohydrates 3.5g; fat 10.2g; sodium 48.5mg.

SPICY RANCH CAULIFLOWER CRACKERS

Prep:
20 mins
Cook:
35 mins
Additional:
15 mins
Total:
1 hr 10 mins
Servings:
18
Yield:
18 crackers

INGREDIENTS:

1 (12 ounce) package frozen riced cauliflower
cheese cloth
1 egg
1 tablespoon dry ranch salad dressing mix
⅛ teaspoon cayenne pepper, or more to taste
1 cup shredded Parmesan cheese

DIRECTIONS:

1

Place riced cauliflower in a microwave-safe bowl. Microwave, covered, for 3 to 4 minutes. Transfer to a cheesecloth-lined strainer and allow to cool for 15 minutes. Squeeze moisture out of the cooled riced cauliflower.

2

Preheat the oven to 425 degrees F (220 degrees C). Line a baking sheet with parchment paper.

3

Combine riced cauliflower, egg, ranch mix, and cayenne pepper in a bowl and mix well. Stir in Parmesan cheese until incorporated.

4

Drop mixture with a small cookie scoop onto the prepared cookie sheet and flatten with a small hand rolling pin, a cup, or your hand to approximately 1/16-inch thickness. The thinner the dough, the crispier the cracker.

5

Bake crackers in the preheated oven for 10 minutes, flip, and bake for an additional 10 minutes. Cool on a wire rack.

NUTRITION FACTS:

29 calories; protein 2.5g; carbohydrates 1.3g; fat 1.5g; cholesterol 14.2mg; sodium 103.5mg.

SIMPLE BRITISH FLAPJACK

Prep:
15 mins
Cook:
15 mins
Total:
30 mins
Servings:
8
Yield:
8 servings

INGREDIENTS:

½ cup butter
3 tablespoons white sugar
2 tablespoons golden syrup
2 cups rolled oats
5 tablespoons raisins (Optional)
1 (5 ounce) milk chocolate, melted (Optional)

DIRECTIONS:

1

Preheat the oven to 350 degrees F (175 degrees C). Lightly butter a baking pan.

2

Combine butter, sugar, and golden syrup in a saucepan over low heat. Mix until butter has melted and sugar has dissolved. Remove from heat. Add 2 cups oats and raisins. Mix until oats are well coated. Pour mixture into the prepared pan; flatten down with the back of a spoon.

3

Bake in the preheated oven until golden brown on top, 10 to 20 minutes. Let flapjack cool.

4

Melt chocolate in a microwave-safe glass or ceramic bowl in 15-second intervals, stirring after each interval, 1 to 3 minutes. Pour over the cooled flapjack. Let cool until chocolate is set.

NUTRITION FACTS:

330 calories; protein 4.4g; carbohydrates 38.5g; fat 18.4g; cholesterol 34.8mg; sodium 101.6mg.

BACON-BLEU CHEESE BALL

Prep:
10 mins
Additional:
3 hrs
Total:
3 hrs 10 mins
Servings:
20
Yield:
20 servings

INGREDIENTS:

2 (8 ounce) packages cream cheese, softened
1 (3 ounce) package bacon bits (such as Oscar Mayer®)
3 ounces crumbled blue cheese
¼ cup blue cheese salad dressing, or to taste
2 green onions, chopped
½ teaspoon garlic powder
¼ cup dried parsley, or as needed (Optional)

DIRECTIONS:

1

Stir cream cheese, bacon bits, blue cheese, salad dressing, green onions, and garlic powder together in a bowl. Form mixture into 2 balls, cover each with plastic wrap, and refrigerate
until chilled and firm, 3 hours or overnight.

2

Remove cheese balls from plastic wrap and roll in parsley.

NUTRITION FACTS:

125 calories; protein 4.6g; carbohydrates 1.2g; fat 11.6g; cholesterol 31.4mg; sodium 292.6mg.

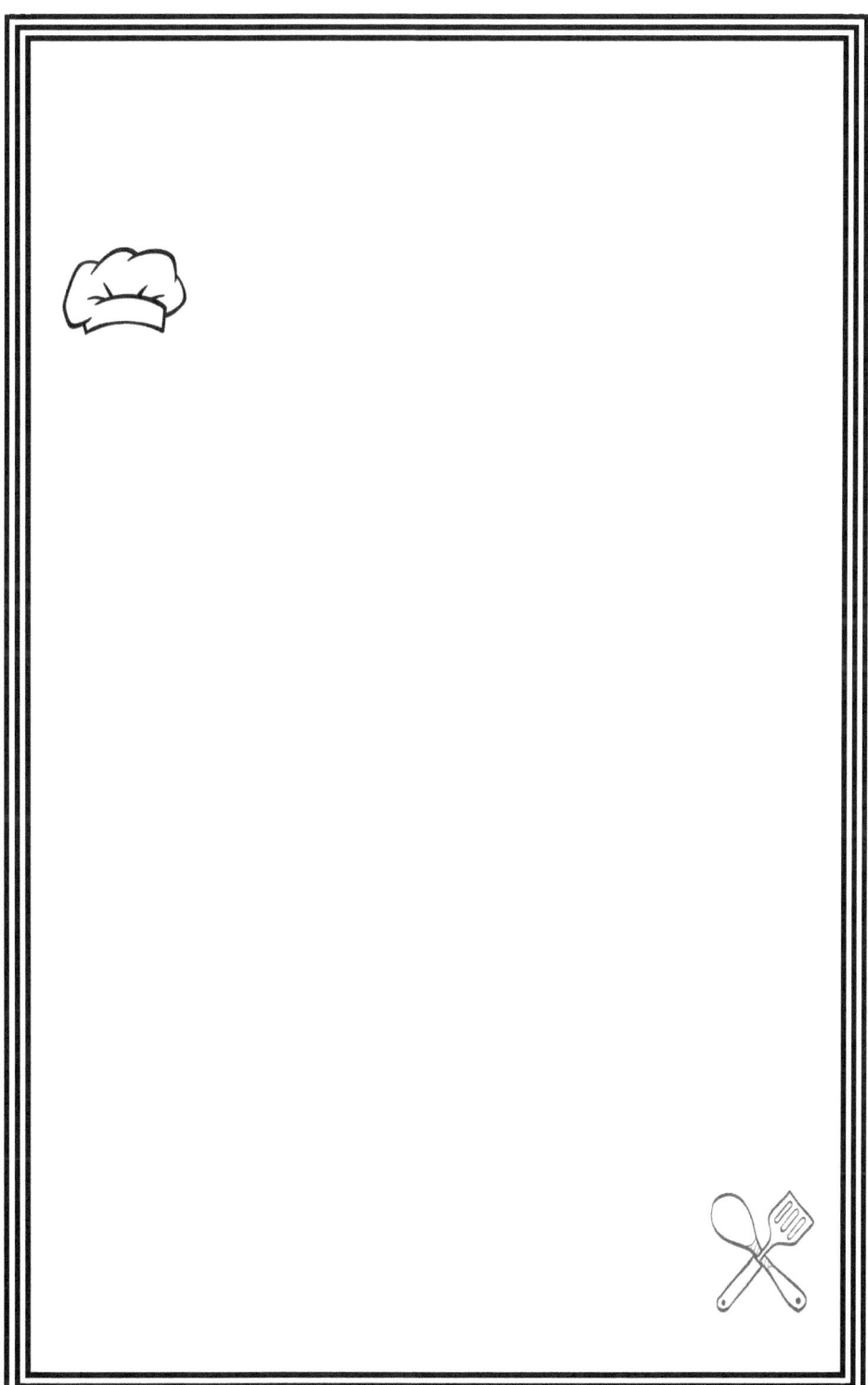

CHAPTER 6: POULTRY RECIPES

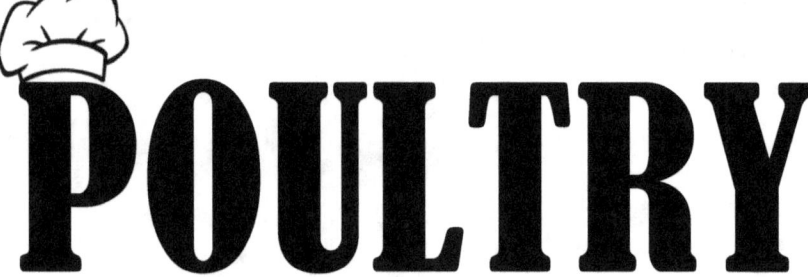

CHICKEN PAPRIKA

Prep:
20 mins
Cook:
20 mins
Total:
40 mins
Servings:
12
Yield:
12 servings

INGREDIENTS:

⅓ cup all-purpose flour
2 tablespoons paprika
1 teaspoon salt
1 pinch ground black pepper
6 skinless, boneless chicken breast halves, cut into bite-size pieces
2 tablespoons vegetable oil
1 onion, chopped
4 cloves garlic, minced
1 cup chicken stock
2 tablespoons tomato paste
1 ½ cups sour cream
1 tablespoon paprika
1 teaspoon cornstarch

DIRECTIONS:

1

Mix flour, 2 tablespoons paprika, salt, and pepper on a shallow plate. Dip chicken pieces in mixture to coat.

2

Heat vegetable oil in a heavy skillet over medium heat. Cook and stir chicken in hot oil until browned completely, about 5 minutes. Remove chicken with a slotted spoon to a bowl, reserving oil and drippings in skillet.

3

Cook and stir onion and garlic in the reserved drippings until tender, about 5 minutes. Return chicken to the skillet. Pour chicken stock over the chicken mixture. Stir tomato paste into the chicken stock until integrated completely.

4

Bring the chicken stock to a boil, reduce heat to medium-low, place a cover on the skillet, and cook at a simmer until the chicken is cooked through, 5 to 8 minutes.

5

Whisk sour cream, 1 teaspoon paprika, and cornstarch together in a small bowl; stir into the chicken mixture and cook until hot, 2 to 3 minutes.

NUTRITION FACTS:

170 calories; protein 13g; carbohydrates 7.8g; fat 9.8g; cholesterol 42mg;

PRETZEL CHICKEN DIPPERS

Prep:
10 mins
Additional:
20 mins
Total:
30 mins
Servings:
12
Yield:
12 servings

INGREDIENTS:

1 ½ pounds boneless skinless chicken breasts, cut into 1-1/2 to 2-inch pieces
1 packet Crunchy Pretzel Flavor Seasoned Coating Mix
¼ pound VELVEETA, cut into 1/2-inch cubes
3 tablespoons milk
1 teaspoon GREY POUPON Dijon Mustard

DIRECTIONS:

1
Heat oven to 400 degrees F.

2
Coat chicken with coating
mix and bake as directed on package.

3
Microwave remaining ingredients in microwaveable bowl on HIGH 1 to 1-1/2 min. or until VELVEETA is completely melted and sauce is well blended, stirring after 1 min.

4
Serve chicken with sauce.

NUTRITION FACTS:

102 calories; protein 13.8g; carbohydrates 2.8g; fat 3.5g; cholesterol 40.1mg; sodium 273.1mg.

CHICKEN KABOBS

Prep:
15 mins
Cook:
15 mins
Total:
30 mins
Servings:
4
Yield:
4 servings

INGREDIENTS:

4 skinless, boneless chicken breast halves - cubed
1 large green bell pepper, cut into 2 inch pieces
1 onion, cut into wedges
1 large red bell pepper, cut into 2 inch pieces
1 cup barbeque sauce
Skewers

DIRECTIONS:

1

Preheat grill for high heat.

2

Thread the chicken, green bell pepper, onion, and red bell pepper pieces onto skewers alternately.

3

Lightly oil the grill grate. Place kabobs on the prepared grill, and brush with barbeque sauce. Cook, turning and brushing with barbeque sauce frequently, for 15 minutes, or until chicken juices run clear.

NUTRITION FACTS:

256 calories; protein 25.6g; carbohydrates 29.6g; fat 3.2g; cholesterol 67.2mg;

www.ingramcontent.com/pod-product-compliance
Lightning Source LLC
Chambersburg PA
CBHW070930080526
44589CB00013B/1467